50 Things to Know Before Going on a Hike

I0438412

A Beginner's Guide To A Safe and Meaningful Outdoors Experience

Jonai Republica

Jonai Republica

Order Information: To order this title please email lbrenenc@gmail.com or visit GreaterThanATourist.com. A bulk discount can be provided.

Cover Template Creator: Lisa Rusczyk Ed. D. using Canva.
Cover Creator: Lisa Rusczyk Ed. D.
Image: Brewed Photo by Jade Dhury

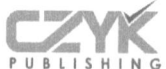

Lock Haven, PA

ISBN: 9781549649073

50 Things to Know Before Going on a Hike

BOOK DESCRIPTION

Do you want to try hiking but fear getting injured, lost or worn out?

Do you want to know how to maximize the benefits of going outdoors?

Are you looking for a beginner-friendly guide to help you make your trip safer, enjoyable, meaningful yet less tiring?

If you answered yes to any of these questions, then this book is for you...

50 Things To Know Before Going On A Hike by Jonai Republica offers an approach to help you be prepared enough to have a fun, safe and meaningful hike.

Most books on hiking tells you the authors' trail stories, mishaps and lessons learned during their own grand adventures, as well as tips on the best gears to bring.

Although there's nothing wrong with that, it is equally important for beginners to know what to do before and during the hike to make the best out of the experience.

Based on knowledge from the world's leading experts, the best outdoors experience comes to those who are prepared.

In these pages you'll find a combination of planning guides, preparation and packing tips, hiking techniques, and life lessons that others only have known by experience after they have suffered the consequence of ignorance.

This book will help you prepare logistically, physically, mentally and spiritually before you hit the trail.

By the time you finish this book, you will know everything you need to know to have a successful and memorable hike.

So grab YOUR copy today. You'll be glad you did.

For each 50 Things to Know book that is sold (not including free days), 10 cents is given to teaching and learning. Go to 50ThingsToKnow.com/GivingBack to find out more.

TABLE OF CONTENTS

Jonai Republica

DEDICATION

To the One who created our breathtaking Earth.

Jonai Republica

ABOUT THE AUTHOR

A freelance blogger and an outdoor enthusiast, Jonai Republica discovered her passion for hiking when she joined a group of couch surfers from different countries in a hiking adventure to the crater of Taal Volcano in the Philippines. She, along with these travelers, founded The Wanderwalkers, a growing travel group existing to include first-timers in its hiking events. She has organized hiking events in her own country The Philippines, as well as in Malaysia and Vietnam, not for profit but to give an opportunity to others who wants to have an amazing experience with nature. Having hiked over 20 mountains in a span of ten months since she started in April 2016, she is writing this book not just to help readers prepare for a successful hike, but more importantly to inspire them to get out of their comfort zone to experience life to the full.

Jonai Republica

FROM THE PUBLISHER

Traveling can be one of the most important parts of a person's life. The anticipation and memories that you have are some of the best. As a publisher of the Greater Than a Tourist book series, as well as the popular 50 Things to Know book series, we strive to help you learn about new places, spark your imagination, and inspire you. Wherever you are and whatever you do I wish you safe, fun, and inspiring travel.

Lisa Rusczyk Ed. D.

CZYK Publishing

Jonai Republica

INTRODUCTION

"There are far, far better things ahead

than any we leave behind."

-C.S. Lewis

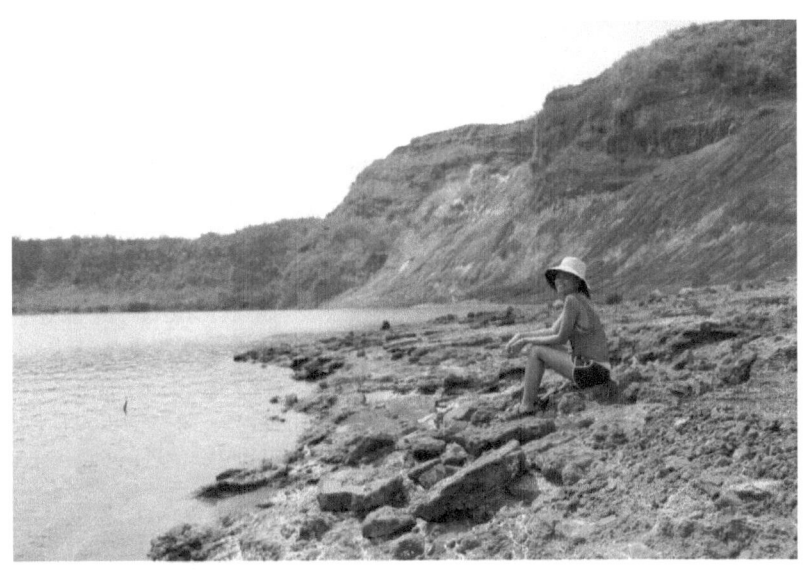

Swimming in a warm sulfuric lake right on the crater of the smallest active volcano in the world is an epic adventure not everybody gets the chance to experience. What led me there, however was a spontaneous decision I made while I was sitting in my office cubicle four days prior to my first hike ever. Little did I know that my spontaneity at that moment would promote consistency in the months that followed.

The trail was grueling, each step on the dusty volcanic path was a test made more challenging by the heat of the sun at its peak, with no tall trees available to provide shade. Carrying only a tiny bag, thinking a 300meter elevation would only take a while, I never felt so thirsty and hungry before. However, had I not persevered, I wouldn't have the chance to reminisce the refreshing sight of a turquoise volcanic lake, the feeling of accomplishing a round-trip trail, let alone the new passion I gained from this outdoor activity.

The countless hiking journeys that followed not only brightened my perspective and made me more excited about life, but transformed my character to be a better, happier individual.

Nature's beauty and adversity prove to be an effective formula in

shifting a mind's paradigm boxed by materialism. Experiencing

this change is not that hard, though. You just need to take the first

small step, not sooner, not later, but now.

Jonai Republica

1. Stop Daydreaming, Start Planning

You've seen awesome hiking pictures in your social media network. You've liked Instagram posts of people with a scenic nature background, and you wish you could have the same experience. You perfectly know that there are weekends you could allot for a more worthwhile activity than watching TV or playing computer games. Now, there's just one thing that separates you from experiencing a memorable nature adventure… your daydreaming. When I said in the introduction that to experience a life-changing encounter in the wild, you need to take the first small step now, I literally meant now. If you wait for perfect conditions, you will never get anything done. I would say that a hike starts in front of a computer when you do your planning and research. Malcolm Forbes once said that putting pen to paper lights more fire than matches ever will. So, kindle your passion for hiking as you scribble ideas while along!

2. Understand What Hiking Is

Let's clear the confusion about hiking, trekking, backpacking and mountaineering or mountain climbing. Although hiking and trekking are similar in the way that both require walking in a nature trail, they differentiate in the level of challenge posed to the participants. Hiking is a leisure activity done on established paths or man-made roads that are also available for modes of transport such as bicycle, motorbike or horses, without requiring navigation assistance from local guides. Hiking trails may include paths established in national parks, hills or mountains. A hike that can be completed in a 24-hour span is called a day hike. Extend it overnight with camping gears and it becomes backpacking, although the same term could also refer to an extended budget travel as opposed to staying in luxurious hotels and booking tour agencies. Trekking on the other hand is more rigorous, requiring extensive walks for many days on uncharted areas not accessible to transport methods. Trekkers are usually aided by porters and local guides to respectively navigate the territory and carry massive camping equipment along. Hiking and trekking can also be mountaineering if the intention is to reach a mountain's summit, although mountain climbing can involve other activities such as bouldering, scrambling and traversing iced slopes. Having said that, day hike is the best recommendation for beginners.

3. Pin The Date

Planning is not very fruitful if you don't even have an available schedule for the activity you intend to pursue. Peek at your calendar and pick the nearest Saturday that you could block for a day hike. This allows you to bring lighter load compared to an overnight backpacking where you must bring a tent and sleeping bag. Although a Saturday means you would probably share the trail with many hikers, it is still ideal so you could spend the next day resting before going back to work on a Monday, unless you have a different work schedule. Once the date is already set, it's likely that you will be more excited and have the initiative to prepare for the hike.

4. Pick A Hiking Trail

Google "day hikes near (insert your location)" to find trails to choose from. In your search results, you may find tour operators offering to guide you at a cost. Although there's nothing wrong with that, in fact book it if you feel safer going with an organized hike, but it's entirely a different experience doing it on your own. Do-It-Yourself hikes provide a bigger avenue to grow in your character especially in terms of responsibility and decision-making. Depending on your location, trails are usually categorized into levels i.e. very easy, easy, intermediate or difficult, as well as trail class i.e. trolling, hiking on a rugged terrain, scrambling on rocks, or free climbing. Start with easy trails first.

5. Don't Let Lack Of Gears Delay You

It's a myth that you should have a complete set of gears before you hike. In fact, you should do the opposite. Try hiking having just the minimum gear first. If you enjoy it too much and feel it's something you want to pursue regularly, then start investing little by little. It's no point buying a complete hiking set, not to mention they're expensive, if you're not sure you're up for it for the long haul. The only thing that is indispensable anyway is your footwear.

6. Read About The Trail

Look for blogs and videos of people who have hiked your chosen trail before so that you have an idea of what to expect. Don't worry, seeing other people's experience will not spoil your hike! Spoilers in movies are bad, but in outdoors, they are good. Going through the actual hike is still entirely different from reading and watching clips of it. Take note of tips specific to your chosen trail, including navigation, transportation instructions, possible threats and required fees.

7. Heed The Weather Forecast

Now that you have a date and a track, check the weather forecast and heed its advice. For beginners, it's best to do a hike on a clear day without the threat of rain to eliminate possible dangers. I have disregarded this wisdom a lot of times as I hiked despite a forecasted rain. Although most of the chances I took were a successful risk, there was one instance when it indeed rained, causing me to suffer each step with my open sandals sinking on a slippery muddy slope covering the entire mountain trail. If your chosen date doesn't show a good weather, either move it to the next possible weekend or choose another trail with a better climate.

8. Prepare Your Body

I know a lot of hikers who don't have a consistent active lifestyle before going on hikes. Count me in. Most of them are stuck in their offices during the weekdays without a chance to go to the gym. Although there's a big probability that you will still finish the trail despite the lack of physical preparation, the muscle pains you will experience during the hike will add to your struggle. You will feel even more sore the days after. So how do you minimize this setback? Conditioning is key! Do easy workouts that target your quads, hamstrings and thighs. Cardio training is equally important. If it's possible, you can bike or walk to work or around your neighborhood. Another easy way is to do home workouts that don't need equipment, e.g. squats, step-ups/step-downs, back extensions and stretches. Do this consistently everyday so your body will not get shocked when you put it under hours of walking.

9. Tag Buddies

Although solo hiking is an accomplishment of a lifetime, you should save it for later when you've gained more outdoor skills. Consider your list of friends whom you enjoy spending an entire day with, and invite them to join you, but don't be discouraged if you convinced none. The worst thing that you can do is to cancel the plan due to the fear of having no companion. You can join

Facebook groups of hikers/climbers around your state or city and post an invitation to any joiners. Members of these communities are mostly up for hikes and don't mind joining strangers. You might even get an experienced hiker to join you to your advantage. Aside from having company during the hike, you might even gain a new friend, and who knows the possibilities?

10. Write And Post Your Itinerary

Most likely, itineraries for the trail you have chosen are available from the internet for you to customize per your situation. This schedule of your planned route serve a couple of purpose: one is to make sure you finish your day hike before sundown, and another is to give your friends and family an idea of where to find you just in case you go missing. This is best practice whether you are a beginner or an expert in hiking. After you write down your itinerary, send it to your friends and family. Following is a simple pattern you can follow for a mountain trail. It could get more detailed by putting transportation elements.

0400 – Departure from house

0600 – Arrival at the park / register/ breakfast

0630 – Start ascend

1000 – Arrival at the summit / lunch

1200 – Start descend

0300 – Arrival at the registration / freshen up

0400 – Departure from the park

0600 – Arrival back home

Jonai Republica

"If you wait for perfect conditions, you

will never get anything done."

Ecclesiastes 11:4

Jonai Republica

11. Make A List, Check It Twice

A hiking checklist for winter is entirely different from other seasons. Assuming you are trying out day hiking on a no-snow climate, the basic things you must bring in your day pack are the following:

Navigation – a topographic map, compass and GPS which are all installable if you have a smartphone. Google maps is sometimes reliable, but there are free apps more designed for hikers such as Map.me and MapMyHike, which also record your trail, speed and elevation.

Sun protection – sunglasses, sunscreen, hat.

First aid supplies – band aids, mosquito repellant.

Nutrition – trail mixes (nuts, dried fruits/berries), packed lunch.

Hydration – water and energy drink.

Illumination – a headlamp in the emergency of an extended day hike.

Optional items are:

Documentation – a camera is optional; besides, you can use your phone. But who wants to miss taking hi-resolution pictures and videos of this epic adventure?

Insulation – bring whatever is light and appropriate for the coldest possible weather. Forget about this if you're hiking on a summer day in tropical countries, unless your terminal elevation reaches thousands of meters above sea level.

Fashion – pack a change of clothes for a fresh feeling after the hike. You can just leave this in your vehicle if you're bringing one.

12. Pack Lightly But Wisely

Every gram matters especially when going uphill. The heavier your load, the faster you'll tire, and the slower you'll finish. The lighter your load, the easier you'll ascend, the faster you will finish. You don't need a big backpack for day hikes. You can forget buying a full blown outdoor backpack for the mean time. I even experienced hiking in Philippines, Vietnam and Malaysia with men who brought nothing with them but water, energy bars and a smartphone! However, it's also wise to have a complete essential. A burnt skin after a hike is not fun at all just because you opted to reduce your load by 100 grams. So, weigh your priorities and decide.

13. Pack Generous Hydration

First, find information if water sources where you can refill your hydration pack are existing in the trail. If yes, a liter is enough to start off. You just need to refill them as you hit the water sources. If none, 1 liter for every 2 hours is recommended. On a cooler weather, however, you don't usually feel as thirsty. So, factor that in, too. You could also bring sports drinks, if you prefer, although I personally never patronized them when I hike as they have the effect of making me thirstier.

14. Bring Energy Boosters

Trail mixes are my favorite trail food. Nothing is more ideal than the weight convenience of nuts, seeds, dried fruits and chocolate, combined with the instant spike of energy they bring. They're available in ready-to-bring packs or you can mix them yourself. Another favorite is snickers or any chocolate/energy bar. You will not even feel guilty about munching on them because hiking surely burns fats fast!

15. Prepare A Soundtrack

Surely the mountain sounds are soothing to the soul… birds chirping, trees whistling with the wind, dried twigs and leaves crisping as you step on them, and if you're lucky, the sound of water flowing in a stream or falls. However, hiking can also be more enjoyable when you hum or sing along to your favorite songs. There are Spotify playlists meant for mountain hiking and wanderlusting that you can just download on your smartphone (try

Drive Thru The Mountains, and Wanderlust playlists). Assume that there's no signal on the trail so don't rely on your data connection for your music. Make sure you download them! What's amazing about incorporating music with your hikes is that even when you are back in the city, playing the same songs you played while hiking will make you reminiscent of past nature memories.

16. Charge Devices

On the night before your hike, charge all devices you plan to bring like phone and camera. Having these gadgets are so useless if they are not well-powered. If you think it's going to die after an hour or so of continuous use, bring a power bank or extra battery. Note that your smartphone is also your navigation and music tool so you can't afford to have it dead.

17. Free Up Your Memory Card

A common scenario I observe with hiking buddies is when they wanted to take a photo or video of something spectacular and their camera flashes the warning "Insufficient storage available" or "Memory card is full." Although this can be remedied by deleting existing contents, some of nature's surprises are only available for a limited time like a rainbow, elusive wildlife and a picturesque sunrise or sunset. Don't miss on these opportunistic shots by being ready, lest you just capture them only with your naked eyes.

18. Study The Map

Although getting lost is part of finding the right path, it consumes a lot of your precious daytime, but it can be prevented if you have a prior idea of what to expect on the road and on the trail. Some hiking spots also have trail options which you should decide on before hitting the road. Plot your route ahead if there are multiple paths available. If you're bringing a car, know where to park as ahead as possible so you don't waste time finding a parking lot.

Getting lost is a fun experience if you have a lot of spare time

finding the right way.

19. Choose Your Footwear

For a day hike with a light load, your existing outdoor sandal

would do fine if the terrain characteristic of the trail you picked is

not too technical, considering it's for beginners. But if you don't

have any, buy an entry level hiking shoes or sandals and break

them in before you hit the road. Never ever use new shoes when

hiking. Allow them to sync with your feet before going on a day

hike.

20. Trim Your Nails

When I organized a hike to Mt. Pico De Loro, a daredevil peak in The Philippines, a joiner painfully lost both her big toenails because as a first-time, she didn't know any better to cut it. With each step she took, her long nails were pressing hard against the tip of her closed shoes. Not all first-timers have to sacrifice toenails, though. Either cut your nails short, or wear open sandals.

Getting lost is part of finding the right

path.

Jonai Republica

21. Wear Appropriate Clothing

You don't need to buy a new set of clothes for your first hike. I bet you can find something right now from your closet. Cross out all cotton-made shirts because they're generally heavy and don't dry out fast. Pick a loose dri-fit or polyester shirt which allows heat to move away from your body into the surface to dry quickly. Unless it's summer, bring a lightweight layer or a jacket for when you get cold. Should you choose short sleeves, make sure you apply sunscreen to avoid skin damage. As to whether short or long pants depends on your comfortability. Personally, since I hike mountains in Southeast Asia where it's generally hot, I wear sleeveless shirts and short pants for a greater feeling of comfort and freedom. I just bring sun protection and mosquito repellant to act as protection, not minding the tiny shallow cuts from sharp-leafed plants that I get sometimes.

22. Tame Your Shit

Having the need to release human waste outdoors where comfort rooms are rarely present is a terrible spoiler. Avoid having to dig cat holes, the only acceptable poop disposal in the wild, by using the toilet before hitting the trail. Developing a regular bowel movement is not just part of a healthy lifestyle, but also a convenient habit for hikers in terms of poop predictability. Eating fibrous food at night will help ensure a successful session in the toilet the next morning. Having loperamide in your kit can also be effective to delay bowel activity.

23. Step Outside

After you've packed your bag and picked what to wear, all that's left to do is step outside – literally and figuratively. Leaving your house to hike outdoors also means leaving all the comfort available to you at home. Say goodbye to a soft couch, air-conditioned room, cold water, shady roof, clean toilet, secured wall, fast internet, everything else. It doesn't sound bad at all, because aside from the fact that you'll be back by night, you will discover an entirely new space where you can grow and enjoy. I have proven the famous saying, "Life begins at the end of your comfort zone."

24. Leave Entitlement And Complaints Behind

As you step out of your comfort zone, your titles also fade in the great outdoors. Here, only nature has an entitlement. You're a mere sojourner in her territory. You have no right or claim over her, nor the people you share it with. Whether you are a CEO of your own company or a coffee tender in a local café, nature treats you the same. As you start to face outdoor adversities, respond in a way other than complaining because complaints clog your potential for experiencing the best out of any outdoor activity.

25. Talk To Strangers

You were probably taught not to engage with strangers when you were younger to keep you safe. However, now that you are capable to protect your own self, talking to strangers could be more beneficial to your soul than threatening. An unexplainable joy would simply start to warm your heart as you say "good morning," "hello," or "take care" to random people you encounter along the trail, whether fellow hikers or natives. You might even find yourself some free helpful tips or motivational stories as you share more conversations while hiking. A lot of strangers I met on the trail turned out to be my friends after we got connected in social media. Some of them I even met again for dinners and hikes.

26. Enjoy Every Step

Unlike living in a fast-paced city where we are used to rushing and anything instant, hiking is best enjoyed when you slow down with eyes closed, lips smiling, breaths deep and mind free. Yes, you have an itinerary to follow but your goal is not to check a list, but to be refreshed by the journey. Slow it down, open yourself up to the surroundings, be in awe of small details… these allows new ideas to arise. In hiking, the destination is rarely the goal. If it was, then you should just hire a horse or ride a motorbike to get you to the end. Rather, the process is the goal so enjoy each step!

27. Take Photos

Most hikers become photography enthusiasts. Aside from taking selfie shots with a nice background, take more artistic shots with nature. You don't have to take a photography course to capture great shots on your hike because nature itself is already beautiful. You just need to know basics like:

-Be still when shooting

-Capture action moments

-Ensure sufficient lighting

-Apply the rule of thirds for shots with a subject. (Imagine a tic-tac-toe board over the frame, and locate the subject on one of the points where the lines intersect, rather than the middle box)

-Don't miss shooting during the golden hour, the time right after sunrise and sunset.

28. Film 10-Second And Longer Videos

Many times, when I was starting out, I regret that I didn't take enough videos during my previous hikes. From then I learned to take short and long footages which I could easily put together later using a software or application. Shoot footages of people in action, wildlife, nature, locals doing their daily trade, your steps, the start of the trail, approaching the summit, whatever you find interesting. Try to be still when capturing footages, else you will catch a headache from watching your own videos. Rule of thirds also apply in framing the action. Then later when you get some time, use a beginner-friendly app like Magisto to put these footages together.

29. Get Dirty

Overcome that gross feeling when touching the ground, rocks or even mud. Studies show that our obsession with cleanliness makes our immune system vulnerable to the slightest touch of Earth. Allergies, asthma and inflammatory bowel disease are some of the possible risks of being "too clean." Hitting the road, though, provides an avenue to improve our bodies' response to dirt. Besides, nature remains to be pure despite its exposure to dirt.

30. Learn About Life

Nature is packed with simple truths that are usually overlooked in a perpetually busy, fast-paced city. Without thinking of work and deadlines, your mind could find revelations from simple actions you take or moments you experience, enlightening your perspective by a notch. Pushing one foot forward could teach you that each step, no matter how small, leads you closer to your destination if you keep going. Regaining energy from a short break could remind you that resting from your busy schedule keeps you from burning out. The unfettered nature of the wild, giving you breathtaking views one moment and troubling you with obstacles the next, could teach you that you are not superior, weakening your ego. Reaching a summit could open your eyes that the best things in life are not material stuff but a fulfilled heart. Observe and ponder while on the trail.

Jonai Republica

Life begins at the end of

your comfort zone.

Jonai Republica

31. Get To Know Yourself

Probably one of the most meaningful results of hiking outdoors is getting to know yourself better. You will be blown to see that you are more capable than you think you are, that despite your vulnerability, you can be courageous, that your sense of satisfaction doesn't have to be dependent on the people that surround you nor the gimmicks that entertain you. A lot of my eureka moments happened during my hiking journeys as I observed the surroundings and my response to situations. You also could see flaws in your character that you can work on to improve.

32. Stay Alive

Be aware of the possible accidents that may happen so you can prevent them. Falls, although might leave you with scrapes alone, are accounted for more fatalities in mountainous terrains than any other cause. Extra caution is necessary especially when descending the trail. Heat-related incidents are also pre-eminent in tropical countries, more so during the summer, leading to nausea, dizziness, headaches and heat stroke. It's essential to resist the urge to overexert yourself trying to push your limits. For subtropical regions, cold and hypothermia could affect a person's judgement and the use of hands for simple tasks. Strategic layering is key to prevent this.

33. Stretch Before And After The Hike

Getting your muscles ready for the adventure has a two-fold benefit. First, it promotes flexibility to allow your joints to move freely and increase your motion range. Proper stretching also prevents possible fatigue and injury. Before the hike, do a dynamic stretch (done with movements) combining knee lifts, one-leg squats, high kicks, torso twists and quad stretch. Static stretches (done steadily) like table and hero poses are highly advisable to help recover after the hike.

34. Check-in, Check-out

Don't ignore the registration and logbooks required in most parks' or mountains' trailhead. Aside from providing the rangers statistics on the count and origin of people who use the trail, it's also helpful when someone goes missing. Fill out all the details required, and leave a note of encouragement to those succeeding after you.

35. Find The Right Path

For experienced hikers, choosing the correct path in an unfamiliar trail is an instinct that has developed over time, while beginners may feel scared to even decide. Although navigation aids like trail markers like paints on tree trunks and rocks, flags or wooden signages are helpful, they are sometimes non-existent or have faded for some parts of the trail. When this happens, stop and observe. See which path has a wider trace like footprints and damaged vegetation. Resist altering signage or leaving trail marks on a non-exiting route so other hikers will not be confused.

36. Consider Your Pacing

Newbies usually fall into the temptation of walking fast at the start of an uphill trail as on a leveled city sidewalk, causing them to tire fast and rest soon. A bad hiking pace looks like this: walk fast for 5 minutes, stop to catch breath for 5 minutes, sometimes accompanied by throwing up due to overexertion, walk fast again, and then stop too soon. A good hiking looks like this: slow continuous walk with some pauses to rehydrate, recharge or take photos. Although there's no definite speed to get the proper momentum as each body has its own conditioning, the art of pacing can be cultivated by listening to your body.

37. Eat Breakfast, Take Breaks

Although breakfast being the most important meal of the day holds true for hiking, it doesn't mean you should eat a heavy meal. An hour before the hike, take a light non-sugary meal like a hardboiled egg which should work best without weighing you down when you walk. While on the trail, pause to rehydrate, recharge, take photographs and admire the beauty of nature around you. For busy parks, however, take breaks off trail to not cause inconvenience to other hikers using it.

38. Take Care Of Your Knees

Knees are the mostly used joints when hiking, receiving at least three times your weight (body + load) on a leveled step, and even more during downhill. To avoid bummer knee injuries, observe best practices such as taking zigzag or sidesteps when going up or downhill and resisting long leaps when going on a leveled ground. Walking poles also reduce the stress the knees receive by distributing the load to your upper body.

39. Watch Your Steps

While hiking, beautiful scenes or interesting things could take your attention from where you're stepping. If you find something eye-catching, it's better to stop and admire instead of continuing without making sure of your next step. Careful and sure footing is a skill that will get you out of foot injuries especially in rugged and rocky terrains.

40. Be Adventurous Yet Wise

"The purpose of life is to live it, to taste experience to the utmost, to reach out eagerly and without fear for newer and richer experience." Although this quote came from Eleanor Roosevelt, any adventurous soul could attest to what she meant. Life on Earth is limited that it can even be snatched from you any moment. But once you realize that your days are numbered, you will be more open to embrace new things, to face challenges with courage rather than fear, to make the most out of every moment. Don't let fear paralyze you from trying something fun! Stand (or sit) on a cliff. Climb a tree. Jump in a waterfall. Scale a boulder. Lie on the road. Do something you've never tried before.

Jonai Republica

The purpose of life is to live it, to taste

experience to the utmost, to reach out

eagerly and without fear for newer and

richer experience.

– Eleanor Roosevelt

Jonai Republica

41. Don't Get Caught By Sunset

Hiking in the dark is one of the most horrific nightmares a hiker, whether beginner or expert, could put himself into. Even when you have headlamps or flashlights, absence of daylight attracts more danger like missed footholds and attacks from nocturnal wildlife. Avoid hiking in the dark by being mindful of your schedule and taking the right track. Set your time limit by knowing the schedule for sunset. If ever you're still on the trail by nightfall, pull out your flashlight, whether standalone or from your phone, walk calm and slowly.

42. Leave No Trace

Abbreviated as LNT, the Leave No Trace philosophy is a set of ethics promoted by naturalists worldwide. Organizations providing Basic Mountaineering Courses also include LNT in their training curriculum. This encourages humans to have a minimum, if not zero impact to the environment. It's quite impossible, however, to leave nature as it is when human intervention is present. Erosion happens, paths are created and vegetation is damaged. Still, the effects to nature are less disastrous when outdoors enthusiasts treat it with care and respect.

42. Take Nothing But Pictures

It's normal to feel the urge to take something home from the outdoors to serve as a souvenir. Flora and fauna are the usual victims of newbies getting into the wild. Although taking a tiny flower, a peace of leaf or a distinctive small rock may seem insignificant, it will leave the trails bare after some time if all hikers will practice this. Photographs and video clips should be more than enough as souvenirs.

43. Leave Nothing But Footprints

The carry in, carry out principle is absolute. It makes sense not to leave any kind of foreign objects such as plastics, paper or metal, but even organic waste such as apple core, banana and orange peels are still litters, not native to the environment. From a small mint wrapper to your lunch remains, all rubbish should be carried along down to the end of the trail. The only exception is, obviously, solid human wastes which should be buried properly. So, it's best to be prepared with a plastic bin for where to put your trash. Carved vandalisms of your name and initials on big rocks and tree trunks sure look cool but they are annoying non-restorative human traces that should be avoided.

44. Dig A Cat Hole

If tips in #22 were not enough and you still feel the need to flush out, knowing the proper way to dig a cat hole will come in handy. It's ideal to have a trowel to use for digging, although it compromises on weight. Depending on your trail, you may also be able to use a stick lying around in the wild to dig. The most important thing though is finding the best spot for this six to eight-inch poop hole so that it biodegrades completely without contaminating water sources and without being found by other hikers. Biodegradable poop bags are also an option to comply 100% to the LNT principle. But who wants to carry a poop with him?

46. Kill Nothing But Time

Vegetation usually suffers from human presence in the wilderness. Little plants and grass are stepped on, tree branches are cut for campfires and bamboo sticks are slashed to substitute for walking poles. Unless in a lost-in-the-wild situation where plants and animals are helpful resources of survival, hikers are encouraged to preserve them.

47. Keep Distance From Wildlife

Encountering animals on the trail adds fun to hiking, more so if you are a photography enthusiast. However, it's best to exercise caution, keep from close encounters and just observe or photograph them from a distance. Feeding wildlife is also not beneficial to these animas as it alters their natural behavior, making them somewhat dependent and dangerous to visitors. I once hiked a touristy island in Vietnam where guests are not prohibited to feed the monkeys, no wonder why a wild one grabbed and stole my bag of chips. The monkeys somehow became dependent on human food, an alteration that could have been prevented if humans knew better than feeding them

48. Respect Other Hikers

Selfish hikers who don't consider other people's experience are a nuisance. People usually go outdoors to experience the peaceful silence nature brings, but loud voices and noises of people they share the trail with can spoil it. Listen to music but do it without disturbing others. Uphill hikers always have the right of way because aside from having a smaller field of vision compared when going downhill, they may be in a momentum of their pace. Get off the trail when taking rest so as not to block the way. Offer a helping hand to another in need when you are capable.

49. Finish The Trail, Reach The Summit

Day hiking is an activity that can be achieved by anyone who knows how to walk (or crawl). I've seen kids on the trail brought by their mountaineer parents. I've been amazed by grey-haired couples conquering mountains. I've been inspired by people with a missing limb finishing trails with their supportive teams. As a beginner, there may be a point in your hike when you would be exhausted, tempted to give up. However, there is nothing great that ever came that easy. You can go over, go under, or go through your hiking obstacles but never give up!

50. Reward Yourself

Surely, completing a challenging outdoors activity such as day hiking is an achievement on its own, with all the life-changing experiences, breathtaking scenes and new relationships. However, it's also fulfilling to be rewarded by yourself, not just after but even during the hike. Grab a chocolate bar when you finish halfway. Munch some snacks when you reach the peak. You can also make an exciting personal reward for each time you complete a trail. List items, from little ones to the more expensive gears, that you would like to invest on for your hiking habit. If you enjoyed every moment of your hiking experience, then maybe the best reward is to start planning for your next hike. □

Other Helpful Resources

https://lnt.org

https://www.rei.com

http://www.backpacker.com

Share Your Thoughts

If you found the information in this book helpful in your life and would like to pass these 50 tips to your friends and family, I invite you to share the book on social media pages. I also invite you to review this 50 Things to Know book.

Feedback is always appreciated, and I would love to know which advice is most helpful. We would love your honest review of this and other 50 Things to Know Books. Please leave your feedback on Amazon. Thank you for your help as we continue to make 50 Things to Know books better for others. If you would like to help edit this book, please submit grammar and spelling errors here. Thank you for your help.

Jonai Republica

Contact Information

Website: 50 Things to Know

Facebook: Follow 50 Things to Know on Facebook

Pinterest: 50 Things to Know on Pinterest

YouTube: Watch 50 Things to Know on YouTube

Twitter: Follow 50 Things to Know on Twitter